What Is an Ischemic Stroke?

Chapter List:

Overcoming Mental Obstacles
Inspiring Others, Sharing Hope
Embracing Life's Second Chance
The Never-Ending Journey

Book Introduction:

In the realm of human existence, we often find ourselves swept away by the swift currents of life, unaware of the impending storms that lie ahead. One such tempest that can strike with devastating force is an ischemic stroke. In the blink of an eye, it can alter the very fabric of our existence, leaving us grappling with uncertainty, fear, and profound emotional turmoil.

"The Journey Within: Overcoming Ischemic Stroke" is an intimate exploration of the human spirit, resilience, and the transformative power of hope. Through the lens of personal experiences and heartfelt narratives, this book delves into the depths of the journey faced by those who have traversed the treacherous path of an ischemic stroke.

With emotional precision and unwavering honesty, the chapters unravel the gripping stories of individuals who have been touched by this relentless adversary. Each chapter brings to life the intricate web of emotions, from the initial shock of the sudden strike to the triumphant moments of recovery and self-discovery.

Join us as we embark on this transformative odyssey, where strength is forged in the crucible of adversity, and the human spirit transcends its physical limitations. Through the pages of this book, you will witness the indomitable courage and resilience of individuals who have faced the darkest corners of their existence and emerged with renewed purpose and determination.

Within these chapters, you will find solace, inspiration, and practical guidance to navigate the uncharted waters that lie ahead. It is a testament to the power of the human spirit, proving that even in the face of the most formidable challenges, there is always a flicker of hope that can ignite a profound transformation.

Chapter 1: A Sudden Strike

In the quietude of an ordinary day, life can take an unexpected turn, shattering the illusion of invincibility. This is precisely what transpired in Sarah's life. She was an accomplished artist, her days filled with vibrant strokes of colors that breathed life into her canvas. But one fateful morning, as she stood before her easel, a sudden weakness engulfed her body. Her world blurred, and the ground beneath her feet trembled. Sarah had become a victim of an ischemic stroke.

In this chapter, we delve into Sarah's journey of resilience and adaptation. From the harrowing moments of her stroke's onset to the bewildering maze of medical procedures, we witness the raw emotions that accompany such an ordeal. Fear, frustration, and a profound sense of loss clouded Sarah's spirit, but a flicker of determination ignited within her.

As Sarah grappled with the physical and emotional aftermath, we explore the intricate balance between vulnerability and strength. Through the tears and the triumphs, she discovers the power of resilience and the unyielding spirit of the human heart.

Join us in Chapter 1 as we step into the shoes of Sarah and embark on a turbulent yet transformative journey. Together, we will navigate the stormy seas of uncertainty, forging a path towards hope, healing, and a newfound appreciation for the resilience of the human spirit.

[524]

Chapter 2: The Race Against Time

In the wake of Sarah's stroke, time became a relentless adversary, ticking away with a haunting urgency. Every passing moment held the potential for irreversible damage, amplifying the desperate need for swift intervention. The race against time had begun, and Sarah's fate hung in the balance.

Chapter 2 immerses us in the whirlwind of emotions that accompanied Sarah's journey through the medical labyrinth. Fear clenched her heart as she was wheeled into the sterile corridors of the hospital, her body a canvas for medical professionals to decipher and heal. Amidst the beeping machines and hushed voices, Sarah clung to a glimmer of hope, knowing that each passing second held the key to her survival.

Within these pages, we witness the emotional rollercoaster that Sarah and her loved ones experienced. The anguish of uncertainty, the fear of the unknown, and the sheer weight of vulnerability permeated their every thought. But amidst the darkness, flickers of resilience illuminated their path.

Together with Sarah, we encounter the compassionate faces of healthcare providers, their unwavering dedication like beacons of light amidst the storm. We witness the profound impact of their expertise, their ability to infuse hope even in the face of uncertainty.

Through their efforts, Sarah discovered that she was not alone in her fight.

As the clock ticked relentlessly, Sarah's journey became a testament to the fragile nature of life and the boundless strength of the human spirit. It was a race against time, not just to save her physical being, but to reclaim her sense of self and redefine her purpose.

Join us in Chapter 2 as we delve into the emotional depths of Sarah's race against time. Through heart-wrenching moments and flickers of hope, we witness the indomitable spirit that emerges when faced with the harshest of challenges. Together, we embrace the fragility of existence and celebrate the resilience that resides within us all.

[297]

Chapter 3: Unraveling the Mystery

Within the intricate tapestry of an ischemic stroke lies a perplexing mystery that demands unraveling. In Chapter 3, we delve into the depths of Sarah's journey as she confronts the enigmatic nature of her condition and seeks answers that lie hidden within her own body.

Sarah's journey took her through a labyrinth of medical tests, consultations, and discussions with experts. Each step brought her closer to understanding the underlying causes of her stroke, yet the road ahead remained shrouded in uncertainty. It was a puzzle with elusive pieces, leaving her and her loved ones grappling with questions that seemed to have no easy answers.

Emotions ran high as Sarah embarked on this voyage of discovery. Frustration mingled with hope, as she yearned for a glimpse of clarity amidst the chaos. The medical jargon and complex explanations became an intricate language to decipher, but Sarah refused to surrender to the overwhelming complexity.

With resilience as her compass, Sarah sought solace in the support of fellow stroke survivors and their stories of triumph. Through their shared experiences, she found comfort and a sense of belonging in a community bound together by the threads of resilience and the quest for understanding.

As we immerse ourselves in Chapter 3, we bear witness to Sarah's emotional journey of unraveling the mystery. We share in her frustration, her moments of doubt, and her relentless pursuit of knowledge. Together, we uncover the intricate nuances of an ischemic stroke, not just within the confines of medical textbooks, but within the depths of the human spirit.

Join us as we navigate the labyrinth of uncertainty, guided by the flickering flame of hope. In the face of adversity, Sarah's unwavering spirit lights the way, inspiring us to embrace the unknown and to forge ahead with courage and determination.

[278]

Chapter 4: Battling the Silent Enemy

In the realm of an ischemic stroke, an invisible foe lurks, silently wreaking havoc on the lives it touches. Chapter 4 delves into Sarah's courageous battle against this silent enemy, as she faces the daunting task of reclaiming her body, mind, and spirit.

The aftermath of an ischemic stroke brought forth a multitude of challenges for Sarah. The once familiar pathways of her body had been disrupted, leaving her grappling with physical limitations and a sense of profound loss. Simple tasks that were once taken for granted now required herculean efforts, and frustration threatened to engulf her spirit.

But Sarah refused to succumb to despair. With determination as her armor, she embarked on a journey of rehabilitation and self-discovery. Physiotherapy sessions became battlegrounds where she fought against the constraints of her weakened body, pushing herself to the limits and refusing to accept defeat.

Amidst the grueling physical challenges, Sarah confronted the emotional scars left by the stroke. Anxiety and self-doubt cast their shadows, threatening to erode the foundation of her resilience. Yet, with unwavering resolve, she sought solace in the unwavering support of her loved ones and the guidance of mental health professionals. Slowly but surely, she began to rebuild her shattered confidence and find the strength to face each day with renewed determination.

Through the pages of Chapter 4, we bear witness to Sarah's valiant efforts to regain control over her life. We share in her triumphs, however small, as she defies the limitations imposed by her condition. The battle against the silent enemy is not without its setbacks and moments of vulnerability, but Sarah's unwavering spirit reminds us that true strength lies not in the absence of weakness, but in the ability to rise despite it.

Join us as we stand alongside Sarah, shoulder to shoulder, as she wages war against the silent enemy. Together, we celebrate her victories and draw inspiration from her unyielding courage. In the face of adversity, Sarah teaches us that even in our darkest moments, there is a flicker of resilience that can ignite the flame of hope.

[327]

Chapter 5: The Road to Recovery

In the wake of devastation, a new path begins to emerge—a road to recovery, where hope intertwines with resilience, and small victories become beacons of light. Chapter 5 chronicles Sarah's arduous yet transformative journey along this road, as she navigates the twists and turns towards healing and restoration.

As Sarah embarked on her recovery, she encountered a myriad of challenges, both physical and emotional. The once-familiar landscape of her body had been altered, requiring her to redefine her capabilities and adapt to a new normal. It was a journey that demanded patience, perseverance, and an unwavering belief in the power of her own spirit.

Physical therapy sessions became a battleground where Sarah fought to regain strength, mobility, and independence. Each step forward was hard-fought, accompanied by sweat, tears, and a resolute determination that refused to be extinguished. With each small triumph—a steadier gait, a stronger grip—Sarah embraced the transformative power of progress, recognizing that recovery was not a destination but a continuous journey of growth.

But the road to recovery was not limited to the physical realm. It was a path that required Sarah to confront her emotional wounds, to unravel the complex tapestry of grief and acceptance. Through counseling and introspection, she unearthed the resilience within, discovering an inner strength she never knew existed. The scars of the stroke became symbols of survival, testaments to her indomitable spirit.

In Chapter 5, we walk alongside Sarah as she traverses the road to recovery. We witness the triumphs that are born from adversity and the quiet moments of self-discovery that shape her transformation. Through her story, we are reminded of the incredible resilience of the human spirit, and the profound capacity we possess to heal and rebuild in the face of unimaginable challenges.

Join us as we celebrate the milestones along Sarah's path—a path that defies limitations, embraces vulnerability, and ultimately leads to a newfound sense of self. Together, we discover that within the darkest valleys of life, the seeds of hope can blossom, guiding us towards a future filled with possibility and renewed purpose.

[325]

Chapter 6: Embracing Change

Life's most profound transformations often emerge from the crucible of change. In Chapter 6, we witness Sarah's courageous journey of embracing change, as she navigates the uncharted waters of a post-stroke existence and discovers the remarkable resilience that resides within her.

An ischemic stroke had disrupted the familiar rhythms of Sarah's life, leaving her standing at the precipice of uncertainty. In the face of immense challenges, she confronted the necessity of change—an invitation to let go of what was and embrace what could be. It was a daunting task, fraught with fear and trepidation, but Sarah summoned the strength to embark on this transformative voyage.

Embracing change meant redefining her identity, letting go of the person she once was, and embracing the person she had become. It meant relinquishing control over certain aspects of her life, accepting help from others, and finding the beauty in vulnerability. The process was filled with emotional highs and lows, but through it all, Sarah discovered a newfound resilience, an unwavering belief in her ability to adapt and thrive.

As Sarah opened herself up to change, she discovered unexpected opportunities for growth and self-discovery. She found solace in exploring new passions, nurturing her creativity, and connecting with a community of individuals who shared similar journeys. Through these encounters, she realized that change, though initially daunting, had the power to lead her to new horizons of possibility.

In Chapter 6, we bear witness to Sarah's transformation as she courageously embraces change. We join her as she confronts the fear of the unknown, discovers the strength to let go, and finds solace in the beauty of new beginnings. Together, we learn that change is not an obstacle to be feared, but a catalyst for personal growth and resilience.

Join us as we journey alongside Sarah, hand in hand, as she navigates the uncharted waters of change. Through her story, we are reminded of the extraordinary capacity we possess to adapt, evolve, and find strength in the face of life's unexpected turns. It is a testament to the remarkable resilience of the human spirit, urging us to embrace change as a gateway to new beginnings.

[331]

Chapter 7: Navigating the Rehabilitation Journey

Within the vast landscape of stroke recovery, the path of rehabilitation stretches out like a lifeline—a beacon of hope and restoration. In Chapter 7, we accompany Sarah as she navigates the challenging terrain of rehabilitation, witnessing her unwavering determination and the incredible power of the human spirit.

Rehabilitation became a cornerstone of Sarah's journey, a compass guiding her towards regained strength and independence. From the moment she entered the rehabilitation center, she was greeted by a team of compassionate professionals who became her allies in the battle against the aftermath of her stroke.

Days turned into weeks, and weeks into months, as Sarah dedicated herself to the rigorous regimen of therapy. She embraced physical exercises designed to retrain her body, pushing herself beyond her perceived limits, and defying the constraints imposed by her condition. With each painstaking repetition, she chipped away at the barriers that stood in her way, inching closer to reclaiming the life she once knew.

But the rehabilitation journey extended far beyond the physical realm. Sarah engaged in speech therapy, cognitive exercises, and emotional support sessions, addressing the multidimensional impact of her stroke. It was a process that demanded resilience, vulnerability, and an unwavering commitment to personal growth.

Through the pages of Chapter 7, we witness Sarah's unwavering spirit as she navigates the rehabilitation journey. We share in her triumphs, the elation that accompanies each milestone reached, and the determination that fuels her forward momentum. We also stand witness to the moments of frustration, the tears shed in moments of perceived setbacks, and the unwavering resilience that propels her through the darkest of days.

Join us as we journey alongside Sarah, walking hand in hand through the labyrinthine path of rehabilitation. Through her story, we discover the extraordinary capacity of the human spirit to heal, adapt, and triumph in the face of adversity. It is a testament to the resilience that resides within us all, reminding us that even in the most challenging circumstances, there is always a flicker of hope guiding us toward brighter horizons.

[326]

Chapter 8: Rebuilding Strength and Resilience

Within the crucible of adversity, Sarah discovered the remarkable capacity of the human spirit to rebuild, to forge strength from fragments, and to rise with unwavering resilience. Chapter 8 unfolds the inspiring tale of Sarah's journey as she rebuilds her strength, both physical and emotional, and emerges as a beacon of courage.

Rebuilding strength was no easy feat for Sarah. The road ahead was paved with sweat, tears, and countless moments of doubt. Yet, she summoned an inner resolve that refused to be extinguished. Day after day, she embraced the challenges with unwavering determination, knowing that each step forward brought her closer to reclaiming her life.

Physical therapy sessions became arenas where Sarah pushed her body beyond its limits, defying the whispers of weakness that lingered in her mind. She discovered newfound reservoirs of strength within herself, as she lifted weights, balanced on uneven surfaces, and conquered the physical obstacles that once seemed insurmountable. With each achievement, she celebrated not only the physical progress but also the indomitable spirit that propelled her forward.

But the rebuilding journey extended far beyond the realm of the physical. Sarah nurtured her emotional well-being, acknowledging the scars left by the stroke and tending to the wounds with compassion and self-care. She embraced therapy, support groups, and the healing power of connecting with others who had walked similar paths. Through these emotional milestones, she discovered an inner strength that transcended the limitations of her body —a resilience that was born from the depths of her being.

Chapter 8 immerses us in Sarah's remarkable journey of rebuilding strength and resilience. We witness her relentless pursuit of physical and emotional well-being, and we stand alongside her as she defies the boundaries imposed by her stroke. Through her story, we are reminded of the extraordinary power of the human spirit—the power to rebuild, to transform, and to emerge stronger in the face of adversity.

Join us as we celebrate Sarah's triumphs, both big and small, and draw inspiration from her unyielding courage. Together, we embrace the truth that strength is not solely measured by physical prowess, but by the resilience that radiates from within. Through Sarah's journey, we discover our own capacity to rebuild, to rise, and to find strength in the most unexpected of places.

[360]

Chapter 9: A New Normal

Amidst the fragments of the life Sarah once knew, a new normal began to take shape—a tapestry woven from resilience, adaptation, and a profound redefinition of what it means to thrive.

Chapter 9 unveils Sarah's courageous embrace of her new reality, as she discovers that within the realm of change, a world of possibility awaits.

Sarah understood that the stroke had left an indelible mark on her existence. The path she once treaded had been altered, and she was tasked with creating a new roadmap for her life—a roadmap that celebrated her triumphs, acknowledged her challenges, and embraced the beautiful imperfections of her journey.

Adapting to the new normal meant accepting her limitations and finding innovative ways to overcome them. It meant celebrating the small victories— a steady hand that created imperfect but heartfelt artwork, a voice that shared stories of resilience and hope, and a heart that overflowed with gratitude for the simple joys that remained.

Sarah discovered that her new normal held unexpected gifts and opportunities for growth. She sought solace in connecting with fellow stroke survivors, forming bonds forged by shared experiences and a deep understanding of the complexities they faced. Together, they nurtured a sense of community, fostering an environment of support, inspiration, and unwavering solidarity.

In Chapter 9, we bear witness to Sarah's remarkable journey of embracing her new normal. We celebrate her resilience, as she discovers the strength to rise above adversity and find beauty amidst the fragments. Through her story, we are reminded that life's challenges can lead us to uncharted territories of possibility, where resilience can give birth to unimagined joys.

Join us as we embark on this transformative chapter, guided by Sarah's unwavering spirit. Together, we celebrate the power of adaptation, the beauty of embracing change, and the profound truth that within the new normal, there is an abundance of life waiting to be lived.

[307]

Chapter 10: Finding Support in Unexpected Places

In the midst of Sarah's journey, she discovered that support often emerges from the most unexpected corners of life—a lifeline woven by kindred souls, by the unwavering presence of loved ones, and by the resilience of the human spirit itself. Chapter 10 delves into the profound connections and support that Sarah found in the most unexpected places.

As Sarah navigated the complexities of her stroke recovery, she encountered individuals whose paths intersected with hers in ways she could have never anticipated. Strangers became confidants, their shared experiences bridging the gaps of isolation and fostering a sense of belonging. Within these connections, she discovered a wellspring of support, empathy, and inspiration.

The embrace of loved ones became an anchor in Sarah's journey. Family and friends rallied around her, offering unwavering support and standing as beacons of hope in her darkest moments. Their love and encouragement served as a constant reminder that she was not alone, that her journey was shared and witnessed by those who cherished her.

Beyond human connections, Sarah found solace in the companionship of animals—a furry embrace that transcended , offering comfort and unconditional love. In the gentle nuzzle of a therapy dog, the warmth of a cat nestled on her lap, or the flutter of a bird's wings, she discovered healing and a renewed sense of purpose.

Chapter 10 illuminates the profound impact of finding support in unexpected places. Through Sarah's experiences, we learn that support is not limited to conventional sources. It can be found in the understanding smile of a stranger, the wag of a dog's tail, or the compassionate touch of a therapist's hand. It is a testament to the interconnectedness of humanity and the resilience that flourishes within the human spirit.

Join us as we witness Sarah's encounters with unexpected sources of support, and as we celebrate the transformative power of human connections. Together, we acknowledge that in the most challenging moments of our lives, the support we find in unexpected places can become the bedrock upon which we rebuild, find solace, and thrive.

[323]

Chapter 11: Celebrating Small Victories

In the tapestry of Sarah's journey, small victories emerged as shimmering threads, weaving a story of resilience, determination, and the power of embracing even the tiniest moments of triumph. Chapter 11 unfolds the beauty of celebrating these small victories, as Sarah learns to cherish each step forward, no matter how seemingly insignificant.

As Sarah navigated the challenging terrain of her recovery, she realized that progress was not always measured by grand leaps but by the accumulation of small victories—a steady hand gripping a paintbrush, a spoken with clarity, or a moment of physical balance maintained just a fraction longer.

Each small victory carried profound significance, a testament to her unwavering spirit and the power of resilience. She learned to embrace these triumphs, no matter how humble they may appear, as they were the building blocks of her transformation. With each celebrated milestone, her confidence grew, and the fragments of her shattered world began to coalesce into a mosaic of hope.

Sarah discovered that celebrating small victories fostered a mindset of gratitude and resilience. It allowed her to acknowledge the progress made, to shift her focus from what was lost to what remained and what could be gained. Each small victory became a beacon of light, guiding her through the darkest of days and reminding her that every step forward was a testament to her strength and indomitable spirit.

In Chapter 11, we join Sarah in the celebration of her small victories, bearing witness to the beauty of resilience and the transformative power of gratitude. Through her story, we are reminded that even in the face of adversity, there are triumphs to be found in the smallest of moments. It is a testament to the resilience of the human spirit, urging us to find joy in the journey and to celebrate every step forward, no matter how seemingly insignificant.

Join us as we embrace the power of celebrating small victories alongside Sarah, cherishing the resilience that blooms amidst the fragments of life. Together, we discover that within the ordinary, there lies the extraordinary, and within the small victories, there resides the seeds of hope and transformation.

[327]

Chapter 12: Overcoming Mental Obstacles

In the labyrinth of Sarah's recovery, she confronted not only physical challenges but also the formidable barriers of the mind—mental obstacles that threatened to overshadow her journey of resilience and growth. Chapter 12 delves into the profound exploration of Sarah's battle with these internal adversaries and her triumphant journey towards mental healing.

The aftermath of the stroke left Sarah grappling with a range of emotional and cognitive hurdles. Anxiety, self-doubt, and the fear of what the future held cast shadows on her path. But within the depths of her being, a fierce determination ignited, propelling her forward as she faced the mental obstacles head-on.

Therapy sessions became sanctuaries where Sarah confronted her fears, unraveled the tangles of her thoughts, and rewired her mindset. Through counseling, mindfulness practices, and self-reflection, she embarked on a transformative journey of self-discovery. She learned to challenge negative self-talk, cultivate self-compassion, and embrace the power of a resilient mindset.

As she delved deeper into her mental healing, Sarah discovered the power of community—the strength that comes from sharing experiences, supporting one another, and finding solace in the understanding of those who had walked similar paths. Through these connections, she gained insights, encouragement, and a sense of belonging that nurtured her on her journey.

Chapter 12 invites us to witness Sarah's courageous battle against mental obstacles. We stand alongside her as she confronts her inner demons, as she dismantles the barriers of self-doubt, and as she reclaims her mental well-being. Through her story, we learn that healing is not limited to the physical realm, but encompasses the intricate landscape of the mind and the profound impact it has on our overall well-being.

Join us as we celebrate Sarah's triumphs over mental obstacles, drawing inspiration from her unwavering spirit and determination. Together, we acknowledge the transformative power of mental healing and the resilience that emerges when we confront the shadows within ourselves. In Sarah's journey, we find hope and the profound truth that even in the face of the most daunting mental challenges, the human spirit can soar.

Chapter 13: Inspiring Others, Sharing Hope

In the tapestry of Sarah's journey, the seeds of inspiration took root, blossoming into a profound desire to share her story, to uplift others, and to ignite the flames of hope in hearts that had been touched by adversity. Chapter 13 unveils Sarah's transformative mission as she steps into the role of an inspiring beacon, radiating light and spreading hope to those who cross her path.

As Sarah journeyed through her recovery, she realized that her experiences held the power to inspire and empower others facing their own battles. With unwavering courage, she embraced the vulnerability of sharing her story—the triumphs, the setbacks, and the profound growth that emerged from the fragments of her life.

Sarah discovered that her , imbued with authenticity and emotional depth, resonated with others who yearned for a glimmer of hope amidst their own darkness. She became a voice of resilience, a source of comfort, and a reminder that they were not alone in their struggles. Through her storytelling, she kindled sparks of inspiration, igniting a collective flame of strength and determination.

In Chapter 13, we witness Sarah's transformation as she embraces her role as a beacon of hope. We stand alongside her as she shares her story with unwavering honesty, vulnerability, and emotional intensity. Through her , we are reminded that our journeys hold immense power—to inspire, to uplift, and to unite us in our shared experiences.

Join us as we witness the ripple effects of Sarah's inspiring presence, as her touch hearts, kindle resilience, and breathe life into weary souls. Together, we discover the transformative power of sharing hope and the profound impact that a single voice, ignited by personal triumphs, can have on the lives of many.

Through Sarah's journey, we find our own courage to share our stories, to offer solace to those who seek it, and to ignite sparks of hope that can illuminate even the darkest of paths. In the act of inspiring others, we discover that our own resilience and growth are amplified, and our purpose in the world deepens.

[327]

Chapter 14: Embracing Life's Second Chance

Within the fragments of Sarah's journey, she discovered the extraordinary gift of a second chance— a chance to embrace life with renewed vigor, purpose, and gratitude. Chapter 14 delves into the profound transformation that unfolded as Sarah embraced this precious opportunity and vowed to live each moment to its fullest.

The stroke had irrevocably altered the course of Sarah's life, but within the remnants of what once was, she found the seeds of rebirth. She awakened to the realization that every breath she took was a testament to resilience and the boundless potential of the human spirit. With each beat of her heart, she embraced life's second chance with an unwavering determination to make it count.

Sarah embarked on a quest to savor the simple joys that had once been taken for granted. She reveled in the warmth of the sun on her skin, the melody of laughter filling the air, and the taste of every morsel that graced her lips. Life's smallest pleasures became vibrant hues that painted her existence with a newfound appreciation.

In the depths of her soul, Sarah found a profound sense of purpose—an urgency to make a difference, to touch lives, and to leave an indelible mark on the world. She immersed herself in projects that brought solace to others, channeled her creativity into art that stirred emotions, and became a beacon of hope for those who were still searching for their own second chances.

Chapter 14 invites us to witness Sarah's transformation as she embraces life's second chance. We stand beside her as she dances with abandon, laughs with unbridled joy, and pours her heart into a purpose-driven existence. Through her story, we are reminded that life's fragility is a powerful reminder to cherish every moment, to live with intention, and to embrace the extraordinary beauty of the ordinary.

Join us as we celebrate Sarah's journey of embracing life's second chance, drawing inspiration from her unyielding spirit and profound gratitude. Together, we embark on a quest to infuse each moment with meaning, to live fully in the knowledge that every breath is a testament to resilience and the limitless potential that resides within us all.

In the embrace of life's second chance, we discover the transformative power of gratitude, purpose, and the unwavering belief that even amidst the fragments, life can blossom with vibrant colors and infinite possibilities.

[366]

Chapter 15: The Unbreakable Spirit

Within the tapestry of Sarah's journey, her unbreakable spirit emerged as a resounding anthem, echoing through the fragments of her past and illuminating the path towards a future filled with resilience and hope. Chapter 15 unveils the culmination of Sarah's remarkable journey—a testament to the indomitable spirit that refused to be shattered.

Through the peaks and valleys of her recovery, Sarah confronted immense challenges, faced her fears, and rose above the ashes of adversity. In the crucible of her journey, she discovered the extraordinary strength that lay within—the strength to persevere, to transform, and to find meaning in the face of unimaginable obstacles.

Sarah's unbreakable spirit became a beacon of inspiration, shining brightly for others who walked in the shadowed realms of their own struggles. She became a symbol of resilience, reminding them that even amidst the fragments, there is beauty waiting to be discovered, and strength waiting to be awakened.

In Chapter 15, we stand alongside Sarah as she reaches the zenith of her journey. We witness her unwavering spirit soar to new heights, empowering others to embrace their own resilience and to rewrite their narratives with courage and determination. Through her story, we learn that the human spirit has an extraordinary capacity to rise, to heal, and to emerge stronger than ever before.

Join us as we celebrate Sarah's unwavering spirit—the spirit that refused to be broken, that transformed adversity into fuel, and that ignited a flame of hope in the hearts of all who crossed her path. Together, we honor the power of resilience and the profound truth that even amidst life's fragments, the human spirit can shine with unwavering brilliance.

In the symphony of Sarah's journey, we find our own strength reflected—a reminder that within the depths of our being, an unbreakable spirit resides, capable of defying the odds, embracing the fragments, and weaving a tapestry of resilience, triumph, and limitless possibility.

[308]

Made in the USA
Coppell, TX
11 January 2025

44236560R00030